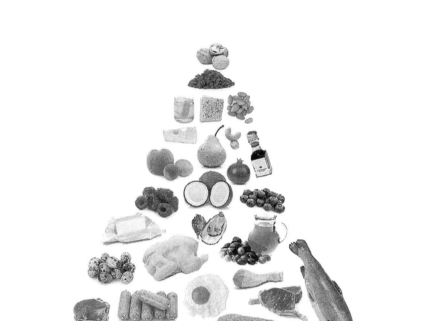

The Real Food Pyramid

Wait! Before You Read On... I Would Love To Share These Free Gifts With You As A Thank You For Purchasing This Book.

Get your Step-by-Step video tutorials to go with your first day of your 7 day meal plan to get you started

Simply visit the website at the last chapter of the book next to free bonus and enter your email to download your video tutorials

Plus Free Bonus

THE ULTIMATE FITNESS VIDEO LIBRARY

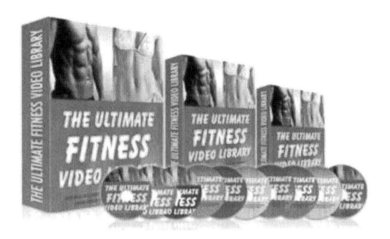

Right now, you can get full **FREE access to 10 video articles about Health and Fitness,** Quality Information that has been well researched, I have put together this Health and Fitness bonus for you because I want full success in you achieving the health and body of your dreams.

Videos Are On The Following –

- A GUIDE TO ULTIMATE FITNESS

- STRESS BUSTERS

- THE POWER OF MEDITATION

- TIPS ON FAMILY FITNESS

- TIPS FOR A FLAT BELLY

- ALL ABOUT OSTEOPOROSIS

- A HEALTHY WORKOUT ROUTINE

- HOW TO STAY SPIRITUALLY HEALTHY

- BODY ART DYES

- AVOID - ACHES, PAINS, INJURIES

To Download Your FREE Gifts Simply Go To The Last Chapter Of The Book and visit the website, enter your email to receive your FREE bonus!!

Extra Bonus

Also included is this **Extra Bonus!!**

Which can really help you along your way to a Paleo lifestyle. You can get access to this powerful e-book even if you decide not to purchase this book!

This **extra bonus** is of great value to you and will really help you stick to this diet. Being consistent with any diet can be difficult, but with the right tools and information, will make your fitness journey a lot easier.

Below is a small preview of what's inside this e-book.

Visit the website below to get instant access:-

http://bit.ly/2DJTvOJ

Strategies That Guarantee Weight Loss For Life

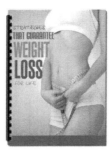

Embracing a positive mindset
Be conscious of your thoughts
Goal setting
Making weight loss fun

Table of Contents

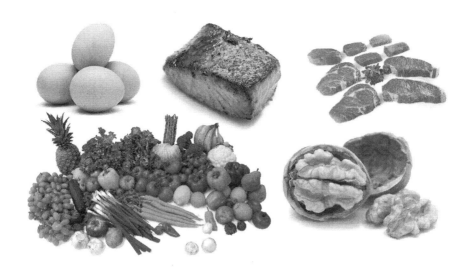

Introduction

I want to thank you and congratulate you for downloading the book, "Paleo diet for beginners."

Do you want to lose weight? Do you wish to lead a healthy life? Are you one of those people who absolutely cannot count every morsel of food they eat or every calorie that touches their lips? Well, if you answered "yes" to any of the aforementioned questions, you have come to the right place!

The Paleolithic diet, more commonly known as the Paleo diet, is a diet plan designed to take you back in time – way back in time!

The Paleo Diet is based on the premise that our Paleolithic ancestor was a lot healthier than the present day humans, without suffering from a lot of diseases such as diabetes, obesity or any kind of cardiovascular disease. So, while following the Paleo Diet, you are encouraged to only consume the foods that were available to humans that lived in the Paleolithic era.

This diet calls for the consumption of vegetables, nuts, organ meats, fruits, roots and meats, while avoiding foods such as grains, legumes, salt, coffee, dairy products, sugar, processed oil and all kinds of alcohol.

You don't just need to avoid heavily processed modern foods, but you also need to avoid everything that humans began consuming after the dawn of the Neolithic Revolution. It was during the Neolithic Revolution when humans gave up their gatherer and hunter lifestyle, in favor of a more settled agro based lifestyle.

But, how can a change that happened thousands of years ago be relevant now?
Well, as Robb Wolf has explained simply: "think of the history of human beings as a large 100-yard football field. For about the first 99.5 yards humans followed a hunter-gatherer lifestyle. During this time the human body adapted to this diet as well as the level of activity it came with. Suddenly, during the last half yard, our food habits shifted to an agro based diet, and our activity level went from hyper active to sedentary (more and more so with the advancement of technology)."

So, while our dietary habits have changed, our genetics haven't really adapted to this change – leading to an overall unhealthy life for most humans! Today, about 33% of adults fall into the obese category, while another 66% fall into the overweight category. And these numbers are slowly worsening!

So, when you go back to your roots and follow the dietary habits of our Paleolithic ancestor, all you are doing is shifting back to the dietary habits that our bodily system is hardwired for, resulting in a healthier and disease free life!

This book contains recipes that will help you kick-start your Paleo diet with ease. All the recipes are quick and easy to make and will not require any kind of "specialized" ingredients to make them! Use local produce from the farmers' market and you are good to go!

I would like to take this opportunity to thank you for purchasing this book and I hope you find the content of this book helpful! Happy Cooking!

The trademarks that are used are without any consent, and the publication of the trademark is without permission or backing by the trademark owner. All trademarks and brands within this book are for clarifying purposes only and are the owned by the owners themselves, not affiliated with this document.

Chapter 1: Paleo 101

The Paleo diet is all about going back to eating the way we should, instead of the way we are doing. It is based on the idea of achieving optimal health by changing our diet to include whole and unprocessed foods that are healthy, unlike all the junk and processed foods that we are used to consuming these days. The Paleo diet is not just a diet; it is a way of living.

Humans have been on the Earth for 200,000 years; we adapted ourselves to whole foods or everything that wasn't processed. Back then, the average homo-sapiens were fit, agile, athletic and versatile. And now the average homo-sapiens are obese, out of shape, sleep deprived and unhappy. Our genetics have not undergone any drastic changes since then, so what exactly is the reason for this drastic change?

The answer is simple, and it is agriculture. Agriculture has been around for a mere 10,000 years, and this doesn't seem to be enough time for human beings to adapt to eating food we do these days like sugar, wheat, processed items and so on. So from being hunters and gatherers, we became settlers and farmers and formed the society we are all now a part of. In fact, the truth is, our body never really did get accustomed to all the foods that we consume these days.

It is no coincidence that most of the diseases that we suffer from today spring from our unhealthy lifestyle choices. And this is where the Paleo approach comes into the picture. It stresses the importance of returning to the basic approach to life led by our ancestors, thousands of years ago. According to this diet, we are supposed to consume all such foods that our ancestors would have during the Paleolithic Era, way back in time.

The Paleo diet works straight forwardly. Paleo is about consuming proteins and fats but also various vegetables and fruits. It is about avoiding the processed foods and nothing else. Anything that wasn't accessible for the caveman isn't supposed to be consumed by you. The human body makes use of glucose for providing us with energy. Glucose is obtained by breaking down all the carbs that we consume.

An enzyme known as insulin is secreted by the pancreas for breaking down carbohydrates and for turning it into glucose. The easiest form of energy that is available is glucose. The human body has been designed to make use of glucose before any other source of fuel for providing energy. All the glucose that is produced in the body is made use of in two ways. A portion of it is immediately used for producing energy, and the rest is stored as fat. When you keep on consuming all sorts of carb and sugar rich foods, there is an excess supply of glucose in the body. This will, in turn, lead to an increase in the level of insulin in the body for breaking down all the excess glucose.

All the surplus glucose is stored as fat in the body, and the vicious cycle doesn't end. So, when you shift to the Paleo diet that recommends the consumption of high fat and low carb foods, this vicious cycle is broken. Your body will start making use of dietary and stored fats for providing energy instead of carbs. This will lead to a reduction in the insulin levels in the body and also all the stored fat.

There are two cardinal principles of the Paleo diet, and you should strictly adhere to them. The first one is that you should consume foods that are whole and unprocessed. Such foods have a higher content of nutrients and are considered to be healthier like fruits, nuts and seeds, even meats (only grass-fed) and eggs, though moderation in eating is advised. The second rule is avoiding foods that are processed and will wreak havoc on your body. Avoid foods that can cause systematic inflammation such as glutinous grains, sugar, legumes and all other concoctions produced in a factory.

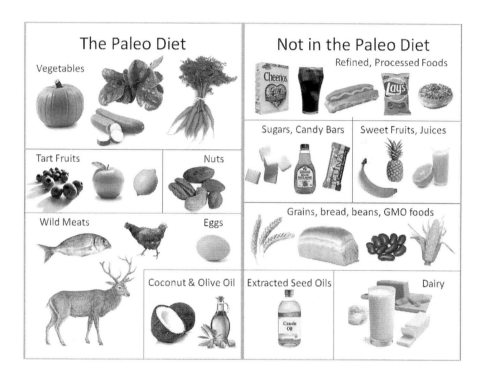

Chapter 2: Benefits of Paleo Diet

Healthier cells:

Not many people are aware of this, but all the cells in the human body are composed of fats - saturated and unsaturated. Therefore, the health of the cells will depend on the balance between these two for them to be able to send and receive messages in the body. The Paleo diet helps in providing a perfect balance of these fats.

Healthy brain:

One of the primary sources of protein, as well as fat recommended by the Paleo diet, is fish, especially the types that have been caught in the wild (like salmon). Fish are a rich source of Omega-3 fatty acids that contain DHA. DHA helps in improving the function of eyes, heart and also the development of the brain. Grass-fed meats and free-range eggs are an excellent source of Omega-3 as well.

Maintain muscle mass:

The primary source of protein on this diet is derived from animal flesh. The protein so obtained is made use of for building new cells, like muscle mass. Your metabolism will improve when there is an increase in muscle in your body. Muscles need energy for movement, and this will enable your body to redirect the flow of energy to muscles instead of storing them in fat cells in the body. The Paleo diet helps in increasing the number of muscle cells and shrinks the fat cells.

Weight loss:

The most notable benefit of following the Paleo diet, beside improvement in your health, is weight loss. The Paleo diet is low in sugar and carbohydrates by design. The Paleo diet prohibits the consumption of all sorts of processed foods. This means that the amount of carbs and sugars you consume will automatically decrease. You will, instead, start filling up on healthier proteins and fats that not only help you feel fuller for longer but will also help you in losing weight by reducing your calorie intake.

Healthier Gut:

Almost all the problems that human beings suffer today are lifestyle related. All the processed junk, sugars and fats are the major reason for inflammation in the intestinal area. When too much of this processed junk is coupled with all the stress, it results in what is referred to as the leaky gut syndrome. Our intestinal walls are in place to ensure that no matter present in the intestinal tract will leave the intestines. However, when this is breached, it results in the leaky gut syndrome. The food is supposed to stay in the tract until it is delivered to the required cells. The Paleo diet helps in reducing this inflammation because it does not include any of these unhealthy foods.

Necessary nutrients:

Vegetables make for an essential component of this diet, and it is advised that you should consume a lot of seasonal vegetables. Vegetables are of different colors, and their colors are the result of the various nutrients they are made up of. So, if you eat all the colors present in the rainbow, your body will receive all the vital vitamins. Vegetables are a very good source of various nutrients including potassium and all the other dietary fibers, along with Vitamins A and C. The Paleo diet encourages the consumption of all vegetables except the starchy ones.

Absorption of food:

The Paleo diet not only helps in better digestion but also better absorption of food. The Paleo diet is all about consuming those foods that our ancestors lived on. They not only lived on these foods but thrived on them as well. The Paleo diet helps in improving the overall health of your digestive system. All the fiber that is present in natural foods helps in better absorption of nutrients in your body.

Treating allergies:

There are a lot of people who have allergies caused due to certain foods. The Paleo diet suggests the reduction in the consumption of such foods. Some individuals are lactose intolerant and others who have issues with gluten. Well, the Paleo diet is lactose and gluten free diet. There is a misconceived notion in society that Paleo is not good because it makes you give up on whole grains. However, the truth is that grains aren't the best choice of food for consumption and you will be able to witness the benefits of giving up grains once you commit yourself to the Paleo lifestyle.

Reduction in inflammation:

Inflammation is considered to be one of the leading causes of cardiovascular disease. You will be able to reduce the risk of inflammation by adopting the Paleo diet. Since this diet condemns all foods that cause inflammation and is in favor of consumption of anti-inflammatory food products. This diet focuses mostly on the consumption of Omega 3 fatty acids, and these fatty acids are anti-inflammatory in nature. The vegetables and grass fed/pasteurized meats and seafood, all recommended by this diet have a high proportion of Omega 3 fatty acids, and this diet encourages this. Omega 3 fatty acids help in reducing the risk of various chronic diseases like arthritis, asthma and various other problems related to the heart.

Better energy levels:

Who would not want to have a little bit of more energy to get through their day of work? The breakfast consumed by an average individual would be laden with sugar, caffeine and some form of carbohydrates. All this will not only make you diabetic, but it will also mess with your levels of insulin, and it will not satiate your hunger. The Paleo diet will help you pick out the right foods for any given occasion.

Reduction in insulin levels:

Your body has a threshold for the amount of energy that it requires for getting through the day. Once you have reached that limit, your body will stop allowing this to enter the energy cells and it will get stored in the fat cells. If you keep feeding your body all manner of processed sugary foods, your body will take the amount of energy that it requires from these foods and then store the rest as fat. If you consume food according to the Paleo diet, your blood pressure and tolerance for glucose will increase and the secretion of insulin decreases, and it improves the sensitivity of the insulin produced, which helps in losing weight.

Improvement in overall health:

It would be unfair to call the Paleo diet the perfect diet, but its main objective - like other diets - is not the reduction of weight. But it is the improvement of your health. It is all about reducing the consumption of those foods that will likely increase your risk of being susceptible to disease. The simple blueprint provided by the Paleo diet helps you cut down on the junk you throw into your system. Eat what the caveman did, and nothing else. If the caveman could not eat it, then neither can you. This diet will reduce the risk of contracting disease because you will be made to consume only whole and healthy foods, full of nutrition.

Shrinks fat cells:

The Paleo diet is all about shrinking the fat cells. Whenever the body has excess energy from foods, it will store these foods in the fat cells. You might not have realized this yet, but your body has fat cells, and these fat cells compress and expand according to what you consume. A lean person has fat cells as well; it's just that these fat cells are small. If you want to keep your fat cells small, then consume foods that are healthy and reduce your carbohydrate intake. If you are sensitive towards insulin, there are healthy fats that are readily available packed between the other cells. The Paleo diet works in improving the synergy in your body. This diet encourages you to eat those foods that are high in protein, and this will keep you sensitive towards insulin thereby keeping your fat cells compact.

Chapter 3: Paleo Breakfast Recipes

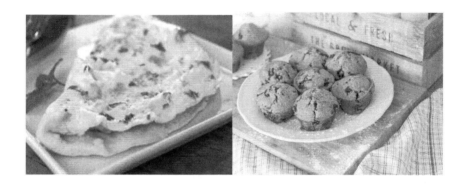

Breakfast Casserole

Serves: 4

Ingredients:

- 8 eggs, whisked
- 1 medium sweet potato, shredded
- 1/2 pound chorizo
- 1 1/2 tablespoon Sriracha sauce
- 1 medium yellow onion, diced
- 3/4 teaspoon onion powder
- 3/4 teaspoon garlic powder
- Freshly ground pepper powder
- Salt as per taste

Method:

1. Place a <u>skillet</u> over medium heat. Add chorizo and cook until it crumbles. Remove from heat and set aside.
2. Add chorizo, and rest of the ingredients to the bowl of whisked eggs. Whisk well.
3. Pour into a greased baking dish.
4. Bake in a preheated oven at 300 degree F for 20 minutes or until set. Let it remain in the oven for 10 minutes before serving.

Paleo Frittata

Serves: 3

Ingredients:

- 6 large eggs
- 4 bacon slices, chopped into small chunks
- 1 sized onions, thinly sliced
- 2 ounce baby spinach leaves
- 2 medium ripe tomato, thinly sliced
- 2 teaspoon homemade mustard
- Fresh basil leaves for garnishing
- 1 tablespoon olive oil
- Sea salt to taste
- Pepper powder to taste

Method:

1. Whisk eggs. Add sea salt and pepper powder.
2. Heat olive oil in an ovenproof skillet. Add onions and bacon and sauté until the onions are golden brown.
3. Add spinach and sauté until the spinach wilts.
4. Pour the egg mixture over the onion mixture. Cook for about a minute.
5. Sprinkle tomatoes on top of the egg layer. When the sides are cooked and the middle undercooked, place the skillet in a preheated oven to 350 degree F.
6. Bake for around 30 minutes until the top is golden brown.
7. Garnish with fresh basil leaves.

Coconut Flour Pancakes

Serves: 3

Ingredients:

- 4 tablespoons <u>extra virgin coconut oil</u>
- 2 tablespoons
- 6 large eggs
- ½ cup coconut milk
- 1 teaspoon vanilla extract
- ½ cup coconut flour, sifted
- ½ teaspoon cream of tartar
- ¼ teaspoon baking soda
- ¼ teaspoon sea salt

Method:

1. In a bowl add coconut oil and honey. Mix well to a creamy texture.
2. Add one egg at a time. Whisk well until smooth
3. Add coconut flour. Mix until smooth.
4. Add cream of tartar, baking soda and salt. Fold. Do not over mix at this stage
5. Add a little butter to a <u>non-stick pan</u>. Pour about a tablespoon of batter (you can increase the batter if you want bigger sized pancakes). Cook until brown. Flip side. Cook the other side too.
6. Serve hot with <u>raw honey</u>.

Blueberry Muffins Paleo Style

Serves: 2

Ingredients:

- 2 eggs
- 2 cups blanched almond flour
- 4 tablespoons raw honey
- ¼ teaspoon baking soda
- ¼ cup coconut oil, melted
- 1 cup full fat coconut milk
- ½ cup fresh blueberries
- 1/8 teaspoon salt
- 2 teaspoons vanilla extract
- ½ cup nuts of your choice, chopped (optional)
- 2/3 cup dark chocolate chips (optional)

Method:

1. Mix together in a bowl, almond flour, salt and baking soda.
2. Add honey, coconut milk, eggs and coconut oil to another bowl and whisk well. Pour into the bowl of flour and mix well. It should not be over mixed.
3. Add blueberries and fold gently.
4. Line muffin molds with paper baking cups. Fill batter up to ¾.
5. Bake in a preheated oven at 350° F for about 20 minutes or a toothpick when inserted in the center of the muffin comes out clean.
6. Cool on a wire rack. Cool completely and discard the paper cups and serve.
7. The left over muffins can be packed in an airtight container and stored in the refrigerator.

Green Tea Very Berry Smoothie

Serves: 4

Ingredients:

- 1 cup frozen cranberries
- 1/2 cup frozen blueberries
- 10 frozen whole strawberries
- 1 cup frozen blackberries
- 2 ripe bananas, sliced
- 1 cup almond milk
- 1 cup brewed green tea, cooled
- 4 tablespoons honey or agave nectar

Method:

1. Add all the ingredients to a <u>blender</u> and blend until smooth.
2. Pour into glasses and serve with ice.

Paleo Dry Fruit Cereal Mix

Serves: 12-15

Ingredients:

- 4 cups flaked coconut
- 1 cup walnuts, chopped
- 1 cup hemp seeds
- 1 cup almonds, chopped
- 2 teaspoons ground cinnamon
- Unsweetened milk of your choice

Method:

1. Line a cookie sheet with baking paper and spread the coconut flakes over it.
2. Bake in a preheated oven at 300° F for about 5 minutes. Keep a watch over the oven. Mix the flakes in between a couple of times and roast until light brown.
3. Remove from the oven. Leave it aside to cool. Sprinkle cinnamon powder. It will turn out crunchy in a while.
4. Place the almonds, hemp seeds and walnuts on the baking sheet and bake for another 5-8 minutes.
5. Remove from oven and mix with coconut flakes.
6. When cooled, transfer into an airtight container and store until use.
7. Serve with milk and fruits of your choice.

Good Health Smoothie

Serves: 4

Ingredients:

- 2 Roma tomatoes
- 2 cups red cabbage, chopped
- 1 red bell pepper, chopped
- 10 medium strawberries, chopped
- 1 cup raspberries
- 2 cups cold water

Method:

1. Add all the ingredients to a blender and blend until smooth.
2. Pour into glasses and serve with ice.

Sweet and Sour Smoothie

Serves: 2

Ingredients:

- 1 small banana
- 2 medium carrots
- 1 1/2 oranges
- 3 cups spinach
- 1 tablespoon pumpkin seeds
- 2 tablespoons hemp seeds
- 1 1/2 cups water

Method:

1. Add all the ingredients to the <u>blender</u> and blend until smooth.
2. Pour into glasses and serve with crushed ice.

Cinnamon Muffins

Serves: 2

Ingredients:

- 2 eggs
- 2 tablespoons coconut flour
- 1/2 cup almond flour
- 1/2 teaspoon baking soda
- 1/4 teaspoon kosher salt
- 1/2 teaspoon ground cinnamon
- 4 tablespoons water
- 1 tablespoon maple syrup (optional)
- 3 tablespoons golden raisins (optional)

Method:

1. Add coconut flour, almond flour, salt, baking soda and cinnamon to a bowl.
2. Add rest of the ingredients and whisk until well combined.
3. Pour the batter into greased <u>microwave</u> safe ramekins.
4. Microwave on high for 2 minutes.
5. Remove from microwave. When cool, loosen the sides, remove from the ramekins and store in an airtight container

Almond butter Banana Pancakes

Serves: 2

Ingredients:

- 1 banana, mashed
- 2 eggs, beaten
- 1 heaped tablespoon chunky almond butter
- Cooking spray

Method:

1. Add all the ingredients except chocolate chips to a bowl and whisk well.
2. Place a <u>nonstick pan</u> sprayed cooking spray over medium heat. Pour batter on the pan.
3. Either make a large pancake or make smaller pancakes.
4. When the underside is cooked, flip sides and cook the other side too and serve.

Sweet Porridge

Serves: 6

Ingredients:

- 1 cup coconut milk
- 1 ripe banana, mashed
- 2 tablespoons flax meal
- 6 tablespoons almond meal
- ½ teaspoon ground cinnamon
- A pinch of ground cloves
- A pinch of ground nutmeg
- 1/4 teaspoon ginger, grated
- A pinch of Celtic sea salt
- Berries of your choice for serving
- Maple syrup or honey (optional)
- 2 tablespoons nuts of your choice for serving

Method:

1. Mix together all the ingredients except berries and nuts in a saucepan.
2. Place over low heat and simmer until thickened to the consistency you desire.
3. Serve with berries and nuts.

Breakfast Special Baked Eggs

Serves: 3

Ingredients:

- 3 eggs
- 6 cups marinara sauce, warmed
- 1/3 cup nondairy parmesan cheese, grated
- 1/3 cup nondairy mozzarella cheese, grated
- 2 tablespoons fresh parsley, chopped
- Salt and Pepper to taste

Method:

1. Take a large baking dish. Pour half the marinara sauce all over it.
2. Crack eggs at different positions on the sauce.
3. Pour the remaining sauce all around the eggs. Sprinkle cheese around the eggs.
4. Sprinkle salt and pepper over the eggs.
5. Place the baking dish in a preheated oven and bake at 350 degree F until the eggs are almost set.
6. Broil for a couple of minutes until cheese melts.

Chapter 4: Paleo Soups and Salads

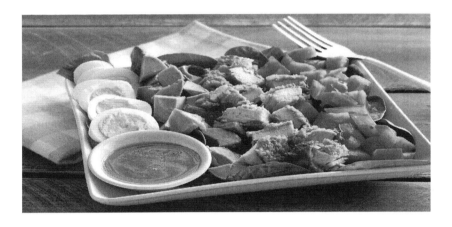

Fruit & Nut Salad

Serves: 1

Ingredients:

- 4-5 almonds
- 1 mango, sliced
- 1/2 tablespoon honey
- 1/2 banana, chopped

Method:

1. In a salad bowl lightly mix the mango, honey and banana. Do not mix too vigorously or you will smash the fruit.
2. Dry roast the almonds on a low to medium heat, making sure you do not burn the nuts.
3. Add to the salad whole, sliced or crushed, to add texture to your salad.

Pear Salad with Honey – Citrus Vinaigrette

Serves: 8

Ingredients:

For the salad:

- 1 cup red grapes, halved
- 10 cups romaine lettuce, chopped
- 1 cucumber, diced
- 2 pears, peeled, deseeded, sliced
- 1 cup cherry tomatoes, halved

For the vinaigrette:

- 2 tablespoons orange zest, grated
- 1/3 cup fresh orange juice
- 2 tablespoons fresh parsley, minced
- Sea salt to taste
- Freshly ground pepper to taste
- ½ cup extra virgin olive oil
- 4 teaspoons raw honey

Method:

1. To make the dressing: Add all the ingredients of the vinaigrette into a bowl and whisk well.
2. Add grapes, lettuce, cucumber, pears and tomatoes into a bowl and toss well.
3. Pour the dressing over it. Toss again.
4. Serve.

Greek Salad

Serves: 4

Ingredients:

<u>For the salad:</u>

- 2 cucumbers, chopped
- 8 tomatoes, chopped
- 1 red onion, thinly sliced
- 1 ½ cups kalamata olives

<u>For the Greek style dressing:</u>

- ¼ cup red wine vinegar
- ½ cup extra virgin olive oil
- 2 tablespoons fresh lemon juice
- 1 teaspoon dried oregano
- Sea salt to taste
- Freshly ground pepper to taste

Method:

1. Add tomatoes, cucumber and red onions into a bowl and toss.
2. To make dressing: Add vinegar, oil, lemon juice, oregano, salt and pepper into a bowl and whisk well.
3. Pour the dressing over the salad and toss well.
4. Top with olives and serve.

Mexican Chicken Salad

Serves: 6

Ingredients:

- 3 cups chicken breasts, skinless, cooked, shredded
- ¾ cup green bell pepper, minced
- 13 cup red onion, minced
- 2 jalapeños (or to taste), minced
- ½ teaspoon ground cumin
- 1 ½ teaspoons chili powder
- ½ teaspoon paprika
- 3 tablespoons fresh lemon juice
- ¾ cup Paleo mayonnaise (or more if required)
- Sea salt to taste
- Freshly ground pepper to taste

Method:

1. To make the dressing: Add mayonnaise, salt, pepper, lemon juice, cumin, chili powder and paprika into a bowl and whisk well.
2. Add chicken, bell pepper, onion and jalapeño into a salad bowl and toss well.
3. Pour the dressing over it and fold gently. Taste and adjust the seasoning and mayonnaise if necessary.
4. Serve.

Seafood Salad

Serves: 4-6

Ingredients:

- 2 pound canned lump crab meat, drained
- 4 scallions, thinly sliced
- ¼ cup parsley, chopped
- ¼ cup mayonnaise
- 2 tablespoons lemon juice
- Kosher salt to taste
- Freshly ground black pepper to taste
- A handful of lettuce leaves, torn
- 1 avocado, peeled, pitted, chopped
- 1 red bell pepper, finely chopped

Method:

1. Mix together all the ingredients in a bowl and toss well.
2. Add more mayonnaise, lemon juice, salt, and pepper if necessary.
3. Serve.

Veggie Chowder

Serves: 8

Ingredients:

- 2 medium heads cauliflower, roughly chopped
- 2 large carrots, chopped
- 2 onions, diced
- 4 cloves garlic, minced
- 4 stalks celery, chopped
- 8 cups vegetable stock
- 2 cups coconut milk
- 1 tablespoon coconut oil
- 1 teaspoon ground coriander
- 1 teaspoon turmeric
- 1 ½ teaspoons ground cumin
- 2 tablespoons fresh dill, chopped
- Salt to taste
- Freshly ground black pepper to taste

Method:

1. Place a <u>saucepan</u> over medium high heat. When the oil is heated, add onions, garlic, carrots and celery and sauté until onions are translucent.
2. Add cauliflower and sauté for about 5 minutes.
3. Add rest of the ingredients except dill and bring to the boil.
4. Lower heat and cover. Simmer until vegetables are tender. Taste and adjust the seasoning if necessary.
5. Ladle into soup bowls.
6. Garnish with dill and serve.

Chicken Noodle Soup

Serves: 2

Ingredients:

- 2 chicken thighs, skinless, boneless
- 1 small zucchini
- 2 ounces shiitake mushrooms, stems removed, thinly sliced
- 3 ounces baby spinach, chopped
- 4 cups chicken stock
- 1/4 teaspoon black pepper powder
- 1/2 teaspoon salt free Chinese five spice powder
- 1 inch piece ginger, peeled, cut into thin matchsticks
- 2 cloves garlic, peeled, thinly sliced
- 1 hardboiled egg, halved lengthwise
- 2 scallions, sliced
- Crushed red pepper flakes to taste (optional)

Method:

1. Make noodles of the zucchini with a spiralizer or a julienne slicer and keep it aside.
2. Rub chicken thighs with five-spice powder. Sprinkle black pepper powder over it. Place the seasoned chicken on a baking sheet lined with foil.
3. Broil in a preheated broiler by placing it 4-5 inches from the heating element. Broil for 8-10 minutes or until done. Turn the chicken around half way through.
4. Remove from broiler and place on your cutting board. When cool enough to handle, slice the chicken and keep it aside.
5. Meanwhile add stock, ginger and garlic to a saucepan and

bring to a boil. Lower heat and add mushrooms. Simmer for 2 minutes.
6. Add zucchini noodles and simmer for a minute more.
7. Remove from heat and add spinach. Stir for a couple of minutes and add chicken.
8. Stir again.
9. Ladle the soup in bowls. Place an egg half over each bowl. Add scallions. Sprinkle crushed red pepper flakes and serve.

Paleo Pork Cabbage Soup

Serves: 4

Ingredients

- 1 ½ -2 pounds lean pork spare ribs
- ¼ pound bacon, cooked, crumbled
- 1 medium head cabbage, shredded
- 2 russet potatoes or sweet potatoes, peeled, cubed
- 1 medium carrot, peeled, shredded
- 2 cloves garlic, minced
- 1 medium onion, chopped
- ½ cup fresh sauerkraut
- 1 ½ cans (14.5 ounces each) diced tomatoes or equal amount of fresh tomatoes
- 2 teaspoons caraway seeds
- 3 cups chicken stock or beef stock
- 1 teaspoon salt or to taste
- Pepper powder to taste
- 1 tablespoon <u>coconut oil</u> or ghee

Method:

1. Place a large saucepan or pot over medium heat. Pour water in it. Add pork ribs and bring to the boil.
2. Lower heat and simmer uncovered until the pork is tender. Remove the pork with a slotted spoon. Place on your work area. When the pork is cool enough to handle, shred with a pair of forks.
3. Place a saucepan over medium heat. Add oil. When the oil is heated, add onions and garlic and sauté until translucent.

4. Add cabbage, sauerkraut, carrot and potatoes and cook for 5-6 minutes.
5. Add rest of the ingredients and stir and bring to the boil.
6. Lower heat and simmer until the vegetables are tender. Add bacon and stir.
7. Taste and adjust the seasonings if necessary. Remove from heat.
8. Serve in individual soup bowls.

Coconuty Vegetable Soup with Lemongrass

Serves: 5

Ingredients:

- 6 large carrots, peeled, roughly chopped
- 2 large zucchinis, roughly chopped
- 6 stalks lemongrass, finely chopped
- 4 cloves garlic, pressed
- 1 inch ginger, minced
- 6 Kaffir lime leaves
- 2 onions, roughly chopped
- 3 cups coconut milk
- Fresh cilantro leaves, chopped, for garnish

Method:

1. Add all ingredients except zucchini to a large pot. Add water just enough to cover the ingredients in the pot.
2. Place the pot over medium heat. Bring to a boil.
3. Lower heat, cover and simmer for 20-25 minutes.
4. Add the zucchini. Cover and cook for 15 minutes. Remove from heat.
5. Cool for a while and blend with a stick blender. In case you are using lime juice instead of kaffir leaves, then add the lime juice while blending.
6. Ladle into bowls. Garnish with cilantro. Serve warm or cold.

Celery and Asparagus Soup

Serves: 2

Ingredients

- 4 stalks celery, chopped
- 20 stalks asparagus, chopped
- 1 medium onion, chopped
- 2 teaspoons fresh tarragon
- 2 teaspoons olive oil
- 3 cups vegetable broth
- 1/2 teaspoon pepper powder
- 1/2 teaspoon salt
- 1/4 cup single cream

Method

1. Place a large skillet or saucepan over medium heat.
2. Add oil. When oil heats, add onions and cook until onions are translucent.
3. Add asparagus, broth, salt and pepper, celery and 1-teaspoon tarragon. Stir and let it boil.
4. Reduce heat, cover and simmer until asparagus is very well cooked.
5. Remove from heat and blend the soup using an immersion blender.
6. Place the pan back on heat.
7. Add cream and tarragon and heat thoroughly.

Hot Chicken Soup

Serves: 2

Ingredients

- 1 chicken breasts, skinless, boneless, cut into thin strips
- 4 scallions, chopped
- 2 teaspoons Thai red curry paste
- 1/2 cup coconut milk
- 3 cups chicken broth
- 1 1/2 teaspoons ground coriander
- 2 teaspoons lemon juice
- 2 teaspoons lime juice
- 1/2 teaspoon fish sauce
- 1 teaspoon salt or to taste
- 1 tablespoon fresh ginger, peeled minced
- 2 tablespoons fresh cilantro, chopped

Method:

1. Place a large skillet over medium heat.
2. Add broth, chicken, lemon juice, and ginger and bring to a boil.
3. Lower heat and simmer for 20 minutes.
4. Add rest of the ingredients except cilantro and simmer for 10 minutes.
5. Serve in individual soup bowls garnished with cilantro.

If you're enjoying this book so far, then I'd like to ask you for a favor, would you be kind enough to leave a review for this book on Amazon? It would be greatly appreciated!

I am trying to reach as many people as I can with this book and more reviews will help me accomplish that!

Visit the website below to leave a review for this book on Amazon!

http://amzn.to/2r432t9

Chapter 5: Paleo Meal Recipes

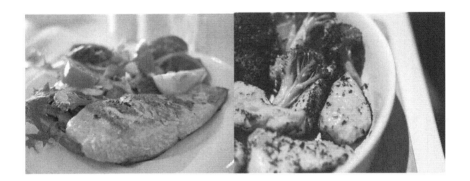

Shepherd's Pie Paleo Style

Serves: 4

Ingredients:

- 1 pound ground beef
- 2 cloves garlic, minced
- 1 small yellow onion, chopped
- 1 carrot chopped
- 4 ounce mushrooms, sliced
- ½ bag frozen peas, thawed
- ½ can tomato paste
- 1 tablespoon balsamic vinegar
- ½ tablespoon fresh rosemary, chopped
- 1 teaspoon fresh thyme
- 2-3 medium sized sweet potatoes
- ¼ cup coconut milk
- ½ tablespoon butter + extra
- Sea salt to taste
- Pepper powder to taste

Method:

1. In a large <u>skillet</u> add butter. Keep on medium heat. Add garlic and meat. Sauté.
2. Cook until the meat is browned and keep aside.
3. In the same skillet add onions, carrots and mushrooms and sauté until the onions are pink and carrots are soft.
4. Toss the meat in the pan. Then add the tomato paste, salt, balsamic vinegar, thyme and rosemary.
5. Cook until the extra liquid is dried up.
6. Add peas. Mix well. Transfer this mix in a baking dish.
7. Meanwhile bake the sweet potatoes in a preheated oven at 350 degrees until soft. Cool.
8. When cooled, peel the sweet potatoes and mash. Place the mashed sweet potatoes in a bowl. Add coconut milk, butter, sea salt and pepper. Mash well. Spread it over the meat mixture.
9. Place the baking dish into the oven and bake for 15-20 minutes or longer if you want it browner.

Paleo Lasagna

Serves: 4

Ingredients:

For the meat sauce:

- ½ pound (30% fat) ground beef
- 14 ounces canned crushed tomatoes
- 1 teaspoon apple cider vinegar
- 2 tablespoons beef stock
- ½ can tomato paste
- 1 teaspoon Italian seasoning
- ½ teaspoon onion powder
- ¼ teaspoon garlic powder
- 1 bay leaf
- 2 drops stevia (optional)
- ¼ teaspoon red crushed pepper

For Lasagna noodles:

- 1 small butternut squash

For homemade dairy free cheese:

- 4 teaspoons arrowroot starch
- ½ teaspoon lemon juice
- 2 tablespoons ghee or tallow
- 1 cup almond milk, unsweetened
- ¼ teaspoon garlic powder
- 2 eggs, whisked
- ½ teaspoon onion powder
- ¾ teaspoon Himalayan rock salt or to taste

- ½ cup fresh parsley, chopped

Method:

1. Grease a baking dish with coconut oil. Set aside.
2. Place a saucepan over medium heat. Add beef and cook until brown. Add rest of the ingredients of the sauce and stir.
3. Cover and bring to the boil. Lower heat and simmer until thick.
4. Meanwhile make noodles of the butternut squash as follows: Peel the butternut squash and deseed it. Make thin slices of it. Set aside.
5. To make cheese: Mix together all the ingredients of the cheese except ghee, eggs and arrowroot in a bowl.
6. Place a small saucepan over medium heat. Add ghee. When the ghee is melted, add arrowroot. Sauté for 5-7 seconds. Add the mixture in it and stir constantly until smooth and heated thoroughly.
7. Remove from heat and cool for about 15 minutes. Add eggs and whisk until well combined.
8. To assemble the lasagna: Spoon some of the meat sauce at the bottom of the prepared baking dish. Spread a layer of butternut squash noodles. Spread some meat sauce over it. Pour some of the cheese mixture over it. Sprinkle some parsley over it.
9. Repeat the above layer.
10. Bake in a preheated oven at 390° F for about 30 minutes or until the top is set and browned according to the way you desire.

Peppery Shrimps

Serves: 3

Ingredients:

- 1 ½ coconut oil
- 2 cloves garlic, minced
- ½ tablespoon coconut aminos sauce
- ¾ pound fresh shrimps, peeled, tails on
- ½ tablespoon fish sauce
- ½ teaspoon black pepper powder
- 2 tablespoons cilantro, chopped

Method:

1. Place a heavy bottomed skillet over low heat. Add coconut oil.
2. When the coconut oil is melted, add garlic. Sauté for 2-3 minutes.
3. Add shrimps. Sauté until pink. Add coconut aminos sauce, fish sauce and pepper powder. Sauté for a couple of minutes.
4. Remove the shrimps and place on a plate.
5. Increase the heat for a minute or 2 and pour the liquid in the skillet over the shrimps.
6. To serve, sprinkle with cilantro.

Paleo Veggie Fish Bake

Serves: 3

Ingredients:

- 1 cod fillet or any other fish
- 2 tablespoons onions, chopped
- 1 clove garlic, minced
- 2 tablespoons celery, chopped
- 1 ½ cups potatoes, diced
- 1 cup Brussels sprouts, shaved
- Sea salt to taste
- Freshly ground pepper to taste
- ¼ teaspoon paprika
- 2 tablespoons balsamic vinegar
- 2 tablespoons honey mustard dressing
- 1 tablespoon fresh lemon juice
- 2 teaspoons ghee or coconut oil
- ¼ cup fresh goat's cheese to top

Method:

1. Mix together honey mustard dressing and lemon juice in a bowl. Dip the fillet in it and coat thoroughly. Place the fillet in a baking dish. Set aside for a while.
2. Meanwhile, place a skillet over medium heat. Add ghee. When the ghee melts, add potatoes and cook until slightly tender. Remove from heat. Add onion, garlic, celery and Brussels sprouts and mix well. Add vinegar, paprika, salt and pepper and stir.
3. Place the vegetable mixture over the fillet. Sprinkle goat's cheese over it.
4. Bake in a preheated oven at 450° F for about 15 minutes.
5. Broil for a couple of minutes and serve.

Stuffed Zucchini

Serves: 2

Ingredients:

- 2 medium zucchinis, halved lengthwise
- 2 Roma tomatoes, chopped
- 1 pound ground beef
- 1 small yellow onion, chopped
- 2 cloves garlic, minced
- 1 tablespoon olive oil + extra for drizzling
- 1/2 teaspoon ground cumin
- 1/2 teaspoon paprika
- 1/2 teaspoon salt
- 1/4 teaspoon ground pepper
- 2 tablespoons fresh cilantro, chopped

Method:

1. Scoop out the middle seed portion of the zucchinis.
2. Place a skillet over medium heat. Add olive oil. When oil is heated, add onion and garlic and sauté until onions are translucent.
3. Add ground beef and cook breaking it simultaneously to smaller pieces. Add paprika, salt and pepper. Sauté until the beef is not pink any more. Stir once in a while.
4. Add tomatoes and cook for 3-4 minutes. Remove from heat divide and stuff this mixture into the zucchinis. Drizzle oil.
5. Place the zucchinis in a preheated oven at 375 degree F and bake for about 20 minutes or until the zucchinis are tender.
6. Remove from oven, garnish with cilantro and serve.

Ham and Butternut Squash Hash

Serves: 4

Ingredients:

- 2 butternut squash, peeled, cubed
- 4 cups cooked ham, cubed
- 2 green apples, peeled, cubed
- 2 leeks, sliced
- 2 onions, sliced
- 4 cloves garlic, minced
- 2 teaspoons ground cinnamon
- 2 teaspoons paprika or to taste
- 2 tablespoons ghee or coconut oil
- Sea salt to taste
- Pepper powder to taste

Method:

1. Place a skillet over medium high heat. Add ghee or coconut oil. When oil melts, add onions and garlic and sauté until onions are translucent.
2. Add butternut squash, and leeks. Cook until butternut squash is soft. Add apple and ham and cook until heated.
3. Add cinnamon, salt, pepper and paprika. Stir and cook for a couple of minutes more.
4. Serve warm.

Grilled Steak with Tomato Basil Salsa

Serves: 8

Ingredients:

- 4-8 steaks (sirloin or top sirloin or t bone)
- ½ cup olive oil
- ¼ cup balsamic vinegar
- ½ teaspoon crushed red pepper
- 8 plum tomatoes, halved lengthwise
- ½ cup fresh basil, minced
- 4 cloves garlic, minced
- ¼ cup fresh flat leaf parsley leaves, minced
- Sea salt to taste
- Freshly ground pepper to taste

Method:

1. To make tomato basil salsa: Sprinkle some oil over the tomato slices. Sprinkle salt and pepper.
2. Place in a preheated grill and grill until the tomatoes are charred on both the sides. Remove the tomatoes and place in a plate. Set aside to cool.
3. When cool enough to handle, chop the tomatoes and transfer in a bowl. Add remaining oil, vinegar, red pepper, basil, garlic, salt, pepper and parsley and mix well.
4. Set aside for a while for the flavors to set in.
5. Sprinkle salt and pepper over the steaks. Grill the steaks in a preheated grill on both sides.
6. Remove from the grill and place on serving plates. Serve with tomato basil salsa.

Roast Chicken with Veggies

Serves: 4

Ingredients:

- 8 chicken legs, with skin
- 8 medium onions, peeled, quartered
- 12 cloves garlic, peeled
- ¼ cup fresh parsley
- ¼ cup lime juice
- ½ cup olive oil
- Sea salt to taste
- Pepper powder to taste

For the vegetables:
- 4 cups crimini mushrooms
- 2 cups cherry tomatoes
- 4 bell peppers, chopped into 1 ½ inch cubes
- 2 red onions, quartered
- 4 zucchini, sliced into 1 centimeter thick slices
- ½ cup olive oil
- 6 cloves garlic, minced
- ¼ cup Lime juice
- 1 teaspoon dried oregano
- 1 teaspoon dried basil
- Sea salt to taste
- Pepper powder to taste

Method:

1. Place the chicken legs in a large baking dish. Add onions, garlic, olive oil, lemon juice, salt, pepper and parsley. Mix well.

2. Roast in a preheated oven at 400 degree F for about 45 minutes. Remove from the oven and keep warm.
3. For the vegetables: In a bowl mix together olive oil, garlic, lime juice, oregano, basil, salt and pepper.
4. Fix the mushrooms, bell peppers, onions, zucchini and tomatoes on to skewers.
5. Place the skewers on a baking sheet. Apply the olive oil mixture over the vegetables with a brush.
6. Roast in the oven for 10 minutes or until the crunchiness of the vegetables you desire.
7. Serve the chicken with vegetables.

Baked Eggplant with Salsa

Serves: 4

Ingredients:

- 2 large eggplants, rinsed, dried
- 2 cloves garlic, peeled, minced
- 4 medium tomatoes, chopped
- 5 tablespoons olive oil + extra to roast and drizzle
- 6 sprigs fresh thyme, use only the leaves + extra to garnish
- Freshly cracked pepper to taste
- Sea salt to taste
- Juice of a lemon

Method:

1. Place the whole eggplant on a baking sheet and place in the middle rack of the oven.
2. Bake in a preheated oven at 390° F for about 30 minutes. Remove the eggplant and halve it lengthwise.
3. Lower the temperature to 360° F.
4. Brush oil over it and place the baking sheet back in the oven. Bake for 25-30 minutes or until crisp and brown on top.
5. Remove from the oven and cool. Leave about 5 cm from the edges and bottom and scoop the cooked eggplant and add into a bowl. Add tomatoes, garlic, thyme, salt, pepper, lemon juice and oil and mix until well combined.
6. Fill this mixture into the eggplant cases. Garnish each with thyme. Drizzle some olive oil over it and serve.

Vegetable Saffron Stew

Serves: 2-3

Ingredients:

- 1 medium zucchini, diced
- 1 small yellow onion, diced
- ½ cup green olives, pitted, chopped
- 2 cups cauliflower florets (bite size)
- ½ pound sweet potatoes, peeled, cubed
- 2 cloves garlic, minced
- 7.5 ounces canned diced tomatoes
- 1 teaspoon preserved lemon, minced
- 1 tablespoon extra virgin olive oil
- 1 teaspoon ground cinnamon
- 1 teaspoon ground cumin
- A pinch saffron strands
- Sea salt to taste
- Pepper to taste
- 2 tablespoons fresh parsley, chopped
- 1 cup vegetable broth or more if required
- 2 tablespoons almonds, slivered to garnish

Method:

1. Place a heavy bottomed saucepan over medium heat. Add oil. When the oil is heated, add onion and garlic and sauté until onions are translucent.
2. Add cumin, cinnamon salt and pepper. Sauté for a few seconds until fragrant.
3. Add sweet potatoes and cauliflower and sauté for a couple of minutes.
4. Add broth, zucchini, saffron and tomatoes and stir. Bring to the boil.

5. Lower heat and cover. Simmer until the vegetables are tender.
6. Remove from heat. Add lemon and olives.
7. Ladle into soup bowls and serve.

Chicken Casserole

Serves: 2

Ingredients:

- 2 cups broccoli florets, steamed
- 1 medium onion, chopped
- 1 ½ cups cooked chicken, shredded
- 1 egg
- 4 ounces mushrooms, sliced
- 1 tablespoon coconut oil, divided
- ½ cup chicken broth
- ½ cup full fat coconut milk
- ¼ teaspoon nutmeg, grated
- Salt to taste
- Pepper powder to taste

Method:

1. Grease an ovenproof casserole dish with half the coconut oil and set aside.
2. Place a saucepan over medium heat. Add remaining coconut oil. When oil melts, add onions, salt and pepper and cook until brown.
3. Add mushrooms and sauté for another 4-5 minutes. Remove from heat and add broccoli and chicken. Stir and transfer into the casserole dish.
4. Whisk together in a bowl, bone broth, coconut milk, egg, nutmeg, pepper and salt. Pour over the broccoli mixture. Spread it evenly all over.
5. Place the dish in a preheated oven and bake at 350° F for about 35-40 minutes or until set in the center.
6. Remove from the oven. Cool for about 10 minutes and serve.

Cheesy Chicken a la Mexicana

Serves: 2

Ingredients:

- 1/2 chicken breasts, cut into strips
- 1/2 green pepper, chopped into 1 inch cubes
- 1/2 red pepper, chopped into 1 inch cubes
- 1 1/2 tablespoon lime juice
- 1 tablespoon chicken broth
- 1/8 teaspoon red chili powder
- 1 teaspoon dried onion
- 1 teaspoon cumin powder
- A large pinch black pepper powder
- 1 clove garlic
- 1/2 tablespoon taco seasoning
- Nondairy cheddar cheese for garnishing
- 1 tablespoon butter

Method:

1. Mix together lime juice, broth, cumin powder, dried onions, and chili powder in a bowl.
2. Add the chicken strips and toss well.
3. Place a nonstick skillet over medium heat. Add butter.
4. When butter melts, add the chicken pieces, red and green peppers, garlic, pepper powder and taco seasoning. Mix well.
5. Cook until the chicken is tender.
6. Transfer on to a microwavable serving platter and top with cheese.
7. Microwave for about 30 seconds or until the cheese melts and serve.

Turkey Burgers

Serves: 6

Ingredients

- 2 pound ground turkey
- 2 cloves garlic, minced
- 2 green bell peppers, finely chopped
- 1 large onion, finely chopped
- 2 tablespoons fresh ginger, minced
- 2 tablespoons fresh parsley, chopped
- 4 tablespoons Worcestershire sauce
- 6 tablespoons tamari or coconut aminos
- Pepper powder to taste
- Salt to taste
- 6 large romaine leaves to serve
- Paleo Bread

Method

1. Mix together all the ingredients. Divide into 6 balls and shape into patties.
2. Grill in a preheated grill.
3. Place over romaine leaves and serve with Paleo bread

Grilled Pork

Serves: 5

Ingredients:

- 2.5 pounds pork shoulder, cut against the grain into 1/2 inch pieces
- 2 tablespoons cilantro roots, finely chopped
- 4 cloves garlic cloves, peeled
- 1/2 tablespoons white pepper corns
- 3 tablespoons honey (optional)
- 1 tablespoon tamari
- 1 ½ tablespoons fish sauce
- 1 tablespoon oyster sauce
- 1/2 teaspoon baking powder (optional to tenderize meat)
- 6 tablespoons coconut milk to brush the beef while grilling
- Bamboo skewers soaked in water

Method:

1. With a mortar and a pestle, pound together the cilantro roots, garlic and white pepper.
2. Place the pork pieces in a bowl; add the pounded mixture, honey, tamari, oyster sauce, fish sauce, and baking powder. Mix well. Keep it aside in the refrigerator to marinate for 3-4 hours.
3. Fix the pork pieces on to the bamboo skewers.
4. Grill on hot coal brushing with coconut milk.
5. Grill until the pork pieces are lightly charred outside and well cooked inside. Or preheat a grill and grill until done.

Roast Salmon

Serves: 4

Ingredients:

- 8-10 wild salmon fillets
- 2 lemons, cut into wedges
- Freshly ground black pepper to taste
- ½ cup minced fresh dill
- 8 cloves garlic, peeled and minced
- Salt to taste

Method:

1. Lay the salmon fillets in a large greased baking dish. Sprinkle lemon juice, pepper, salt, dill, and garlic.
2. Place the dish in a preheated oven at 400 degree F and bake for about 20-25 minutes until the salmon is opaque.
3. Serve with lemon wedges.

Greek Lamb

Serves: 4

Ingredients:

- 1/2 cup fresh mint leaves, finely chopped
- 1/4 cup flat-leaf parsley leaves, finely chopped
- 3 cloves garlic, minced
- 2 tablespoons extra-virgin olive oil
- 1 teaspoon kosher salt or to taste
- 1/2 teaspoon freshly ground pepper
- 7 pound boneless leg of lamb, trim, butterflied

Method:

1. Blend together mint, parsley, garlic, oil, salt, and pepper.
2. Pat dry the lamb leg with a towel.
3. Thread the lamb on the skewers horizontally. Apply the herb mixture evenly all over the lamb.
4. Cover the lamb and refrigerate for at least 3-5 hours. The longer you marinate the better.
5. Remove the lamb from the refrigerator an hour before you grill it.
6. Preheat a gas grill to medium or a medium hot charcoal grill.
7. If you are using the charcoal grill, then push the coal to one side so that the lamb doesn't burn and remain raw inside.
8. Grill the lamb directly over the heat and cook for 10-15 minutes per side. If the grill is too hot and the lamb is getting charred, then push the lamb to a part of the grill, which is cooler.

9. When ready, remove from grill and place on <u>cutting</u> <u>board</u>. When cool enough to handle, slice and serve immediately

Chapter 6: Paleo Dessert Recipes

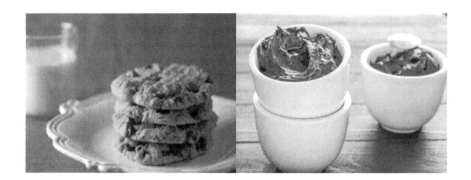

Mixed Fruit Salad

Serves: 6

Ingredients:

- 3 blood oranges, peeled, deseeded, separated into segments
- 3 oranges, peeled, deseeded, separated into segments
- 3 pink grapefruits, peeled, deseeded, separated into segments
- 3 tablespoons raw honey (optional)
- 1 cup pomegranate seeds
- 2 tablespoons fresh mint, chopped
- 4 tablespoons fresh lime juice

Method:

1. Chop the oranges and grapefruit into bite size pieces. Transfer into a large bowl.

2. Add pomegranate, lime juice and honey and mix well. Sprinkle mint.
3. Place in the refrigerator for a few hours to chill.
4. Serve.

Peachy Berry Cobbler

Serves: 4

Ingredients:

- 1 cup frozen strawberries
- 1 cup frozen blueberries
- 1 cup frozen raspberries
- 2 cup frozen peaches
- ¼ cup coconut sugar
- ½ tablespoon vanilla extract
- 2 tablespoons arrowroot powder

For topping:

- ½ cup almond flour
- 2 tablespoons coconut flour
- ¼ cup shredded coconut
- 2 tablespoons coconut sugar
- 1 small egg
- ¼ cup coconut oil
- ¼ teaspoon ground cinnamon

Method:

1. Place the strawberries, blueberries, raspberries s and peaches in a large bowl. Leave aside for a while to thaw.
2. When it is not fully thawed, add coconut sugar, vanilla and arrowroot powder and mix well and keep aside.
3. In another bowl, add coconut flour, shredded coconut, coconut sugar and cinnamon. Mix well.

4. In a small bowl, whisk together coconut oil and egg. Add this to the coconut flour mixture. Mix well. The mixture will be of crumbly consistency.
5. Grease a baking dish with coconut oil. Transfer the fruit mixture into the baking dish. Spread the flour mixture over the fruit layer.
6. Place a cookie sheet in the oven. Place the baking dish on the cookie sheet and bake in a preheated oven at 350 degree F for an hour.
7. Remove from the oven. Cool for a while. Tastes best when served warm.

Paleo Flan

Serves: 4

Ingredients:

- 2 ½ cups full fat coconut milk
- 4 egg
- 2 teaspoons vanilla extract
- 2 tablespoons honey for flan
- 2 tablespoons honey to caramelize
- 1 teaspoon lemon juice
- ½ tablespoon water

Method:

1. Blend together in a <u>blender</u>, coconut milk, eggs, honey for flan, and vanilla until smooth.
2. Place a small saucepan over medium heat. Add water, lemon juice and honey to caramelize. Simmer until the mixture turns golden brown.
3. Immediately pour it into an ovenproof glass baking dish. Swirl the dish around so as to cover the entire dish.
4. Place this dish inside a larger baking dish filled with water up to 1 inch from the bottom (double boiler).
5. Pour the blended honey into the smaller dish.
6. Now place the larger baking dish (along with the smaller dish inside it) in a preheated oven at 350 degree F for about an hour or until the middle part has set.
7. When cooled, refrigerate for a while and serve.

Chocolate Hazelnut Balls

Serves: 10

Ingredients:

- 20 whole hazelnuts, roasted
- 2 cups hazelnuts, roasted, chopped into small pieces
- 4 tablespoons raw cacao powder
- ½ cup pure maple syrup or raw honey
- 2 teaspoons vanilla extract

Method:

1. Add 1 cup of chopped hazelnut into a <u>food processor</u> and process until a smooth powder is obtained.
2. Add cacao powder, maple syrup and vanilla and pulse again. Transfer into a bowl and set aside.
3. Place the chopped hazelnuts in a plate.
4. First dip the whole hazelnut in the cacao mixture. Next dredge in the plate of chopped hazelnuts and place on a lined baking sheet.
5. Chill in the freezer for about 20 minutes.
6. Remove from the freezer and let it sit for 5 minutes.
7. Serve.

Paleo Peanut Butter Cookies

Serves: 12 (2 cookies each)

Ingredients:

- 2 cups honey roasted peanut butter, at room temperature
- 2 large eggs
- 2 teaspoons baking soda
- 1 ½ cups peanut butter chips
- 2/3 cup light or dark brown sugar, lightly packed
- 1 teaspoon vanilla extract

Method:

1. Line 2 baking sheets with parchment paper.
2. Add eggs into a bowl. Whisk well. Add peanut butter, brown sugar, cocoa powder and baking soda and whisk until well combined.
3. Add vanilla and mix again.
4. Add peanut butter chips and fold until well combined.
5. Drop about 1-½ tablespoons of dough on the baking sheet. Leave space between the cookies. Press the dough (on the baking sheet) lightly with the back of a spoon.
6. Bake in a preheated oven at 4000° F for about 9-12 minutes depending on how crisp you like the cookies to be. Lesser time for softer and longer for crunchier.
7. Store in an airtight container

Fruity Sundae

Serves: 6

Ingredients:

- 2 ripe bananas, sliced
- 2/3 cup pineapple, chopped
- 2/3 cup kiwi, chopped
- 4 strawberries, chopped
- 4 dates, pitted, chopped
- ¼ cup nuts of your choice
- 1/3 cup boiling water
- 1/4 cup almond milk
- ¼ teaspoon ground ginger
- ½ tablespoon almond butter, unsweetened

Method:

1. Soak dates in boiling water for at least 45 minutes.
2. Place banana slices on a baking sheet which is lined with parchment paper. Do not overlap the banana slices. Place the baking sheet in the freezer until the slices are frozen.
3. Meanwhile blend together dates and ginger along with water into a smooth sauce and keep it aside.
4. Clean the <u>blender</u> and blend together the frozen bananas, almond butter and almond milk. Transfer into individual freezer safe bowls and freeze until done.
5. Remove from the freezer and sprinkle pineapple, kiwi and strawberry pieces over it. Sprinkle nuts. Pour date sauce on top and serve

Chocolate Mousse with Avocado

Serves: 10-12

Ingredients:

- 2 ripe avocadoes, peeled, pitted, chopped
- 2 tablespoons raw honey
- 1 cup cocoa powder
- ½ teaspoon ancho chili powder
- 2 tablespoons pure vanilla extract
- 8-10 medjool dates, pitted
- 2 cups full fat coconut milk
- 2 teaspoons instant coffee powder
- ½ teaspoon Himalayan pink salt

Method:

1. Add avocadoes, dates, coconut milk and honey into a blender and blend until smooth.
2. Add coffee powder, cocoa powder (retain a little for garnishing), chili powder, vanilla extract and salt and blend until well combined.
3. Transfer into a mixing bowl. Beat with electric mixer with high setting until the mixture turns light and fluffy.
4. Spoon into dessert bowls. Sprinkle some cacoa powder over it.
5. Chill for 5-6 hours and serve.

Pumpkin Spiced Ice cream

Serves: 4

Ingredients:

1. 1 cup pumpkin puree
2. 2 teaspoon pumpkin pie spice
3. 2 cups unsweetened almond milk
4. 2 teaspoons vanilla extract
5. A large pinch sea salt
6. 2-3 teaspoons pumpkin flavored stevia

Method:

1. Add all the ingredients to a blender and blend until smooth.
2. Transfer into a freezable bowl and freeze until done or pour into an <u>ice cream machine</u> and use according to instructions of the manufacturer.
3. Scoop into bowls and serve.

Citrusy Fruit Salad

Serves: 6

Ingredients:

- 3 blood oranges, peeled, deseeded, separated into segments
- 3 oranges, peeled, deseeded, separated into segments
- 3 pink grapefruits, peeled, deseeded, separated into segments
- 3 tablespoons raw honey (optional)
- 1 cup pomegranate seeds
- 2 tablespoons fresh mint, chopped
- 4 tablespoons fresh lime juice

Method:

1. Chop the oranges and grapefruit into bite size pieces. Transfer into a large bowl.
2. Add pomegranate, lime juice and honey and mix well. Sprinkle mint.
3. Place in the refrigerator for a few hours to chill.
4. Serve.

Berry and Coconut Cream Sundae

Serves: 4

Ingredients:

- 2/3 cup blueberries or blackberries or raspberries
- 10-12 strawberries, chopped into small pieces
- 2/3 cup coconut yogurt or coconut cream
- 2 teaspoons lemon juice
- 2 teaspoons honey
- 2 tablespoons gelatin
- 4 tablespoons water

Method:

1. Add gelatin to water and set aside.
2. Add berry of your choice, lemon juice, honey, and gelatin with water to a <u>blender</u> and blend until smooth.
3. Take 4 sundae glasses, divide and pour the mixture into it.
4. Refrigerate until it sets.
5. Now spoon in coconut cream or yogurt on top of it and refrigerate for another hour.
6. Top with strawberries and serve

Berrylicious Ice cream

Serves: 4

Ingredients:

- 2 cups coconut milk
- ½ pound frozen strawberries /blueberries, unsweetened
- Stevia or sugar to taste
- 1/4 tablespoon lemon juice or to taste

Method:

1. Place all ingredients in the <u>food processor</u> and blend until smooth.
2. Transfer into a freezer safe container.
3. Freeze until firm.
4. Remove from the freezer 30 minutes before serving

Fresh Berry Mousse

Serves: 6

Ingredients:

- 1 ½ pounds fresh strawberries,
- Natural sweetener like honey or agave nectar
- 3 tablespoons lemon juice
- 1 teaspoon vanilla (optional)
- ½ cup coconut butter, softened
- ½ cup coconut oil, softened
- A few strawberry slices to garnish

Method:

1. Add all the ingredients to a blender and blend until smooth.
2. Pour into individual dessert bowls. Chill and serve with strawberry slices.

Chapter 7: Paleo Recipes for kids

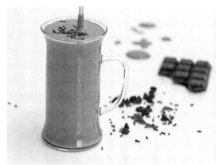 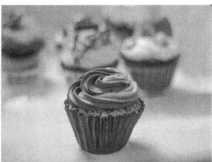

Calzone

Serves: 6

Ingredients:

For the dough:

- 1 cup coconut oil
- 1 teaspoon sea salt
- 1 cup coconut flour
- 2 cups tapioca flour
- 2 eggs, separated, beaten
- 2 whole eggs
- 1 teaspoon garlic powder
- 1 cup water
- 1 teaspoon oregano

For filling:

- Pizza sauce as required
- Filling of your choice

Method:

1. To make dough: Add oil, water, salt, garlic powder and oregano into a pan.
2. Place the pan over medium heat. Bring to the boil.
3. Remove from heat. Cool for 5 minutes.
4. Add tapioca flour and stir. Cool for 5 more minutes.
5. Add coconut flour, eggs and egg yolks. Mix well into a dough. Knead the dough for a minute or two.
6. Divide the dough into 6 equal portions. Shape into balls.
7. Place a ball of dough in between 2 sheets of parchment paper. Roll the dough into a rectangle of 4" x 7" and thickness of 1/4" to ½" thick.
8. Spread some pizza sauce on it. Place fillings of your choice on one half of the rectangle. Fold the other half over. Press the edges to seal completely.
9. Lift the calzone along with the parchment paper and place on a stainless steel baking sheet.
10. Repeat steps 7-9 with the remaining dough.
11. Brush the calzones with whites.
12. Bake in a preheated oven 350° F for 35-40 minutes or until the top is medium brown.
13. Serve warm.

Chicken Nuggets with Honey Mustard

Serves: 6

Ingredients:

For nuggets:

- 4 chicken breasts (about 2 pounds), chop into 1 inch pieces, trimmed of fat
- 2/3 cup cassava flour
- 1 ½ cups almond flour
- 1 ½ teaspoons garlic powder
- 1 teaspoon onion powder
- 1 ½ teaspoons oregano
- 1 ½ teaspoons paprika or to taste
- ¾ teaspoon salt or to taste
- 3 eggs, beaten
- ¾ teaspoon ground cumin
- ¾ teaspoon pepper powder

For honey mustard dipping sauce:

- ¾ cup mayonnaise
- 3 teaspoons stone ground mustard
- 1 teaspoon lemon juice
- 3 teaspoons raw honey

Method:

1. To make nuggets: Add all the dry ingredients into a large zip lock bag. Seal the bag and shake well.
2. Dip 2-3 chicken nuggets in egg. Shake to drop off excess egg and place the nuggets in the bag of dry ingredients. Shake the bag. Repeat with the remaining nuggets.

3. Shake once again after all the chicken is added into it. Shake until well coated.
4. Transfer the nuggets on a lined baking sheet.
5. Bake in a preheated oven 400° F for 20 minutes. Flip sides half way through baking. Bake until crisp.
6. Meanwhile, make the honey mustard dip as follows: Add all the ingredients of the honey mustard dip into a bowl and mix well.
7. When the chicken is done, cool for a few minutes.
8. Serve crispy chicken nuggets with honey mustard dip.

Meatloaf Cupcakes with Sweet Potato Frosting

Serves: 4

Ingredients:

- 1 pound grass fed beef
- 1 small yellow onion, chopped
- 1 tablespoon lard or butter
- ½ teaspoon freshly ground pepper
- 1 teaspoon kosher salt or sea salt
- ¼ cup homemade chili sauce or ketchup
- 1 tablespoon bacon fat or butter
- 1 large egg
- ½ small red or yellow bell pepper, chopped
- 1 tablespoon steak seasoning
- 1 medium sweet potato, peeled, cubed
- 1 tablespoon coconut milk mixed with 1 tablespoon water or 2 tablespoons half and half or more if required
- 1 teaspoon parsley, minced

Method:

1. Place a skillet over medium heat. Add lard or butter. When it melts, add onion and bell pepper and sauté until onion is pink. Turn off the heat. Transfer into a mixing bowl.
2. Add ground beef, egg, salt, pepper and steak seasoning to the mixing bowl. Mix well using your hands.
3. Divide the mixture into 8 equal portions.
4. Grease muffin cups. Place paper cup liners in it. Place one portion of the meat mixture in each cup.
5. Drizzle chili sauce or ketchup over it. Spread it all over the cupcake.

6. Place the muffin tin on a rimmed baking sheet that is lined with foil.
7. Bake in a preheated oven at 350° F for 35-45 minutes or until cooked.
8. Remove the cupcake from the mold and place on a plate that is lined with paper towels.
9. Meanwhile, place a saucepan with over medium heat. Add sweet potatoes and bring to the boil.
10. Lower heat and cook until the sweet potato is cooked. Drain and add the sweet potato back into the saucepan.
11. Place the saucepan over medium high heat until all the liquid in the saucepan has dried. Turn off the heat.
12. Add bacon fat or butter or half and half and mash with a potato masher. If you find it too dry and may not come out easily through the piping bag, then add some more half and half, a little at a time and mix well each time.
13. Add salt and pepper and stir. Cover and set aside.
14. Fit a piping bag with star or round nozzle. Add the mashed sweet potato into it.
15. Pipe over the top of the cupcakes. Garnish with parsley and serve.

Chicken Soup

Serves: 3-4

Ingredients:

- 2-2 ½ pounds chicken
- 4 cloves garlic, crushed
- 2 large carrots, peeled, cubed
- 2 inch piece ginger, peeled, sliced
- 3 cups water
- 1 small onion, chopped
- 1 stalk celery, sliced
- 3 large sprigs thyme
- Salt to taste

Method:

1. If you have a <u>crock-pot</u> , then add all the vegetables into the pot. Place chicken on top. Pour water and add salt. Cover and cook on high for 4 hours.
2. If you do not have a crock-pot, then add all the ingredients into a soup pot or a Dutch oven and cook.
3. When done, remove the chicken with a slotted spoon and place on your work area.
4. When cool enough to handle, shred the chicken with a pair of forks. Discard the bones. Add the chicken back into the pot. Heat thoroughly.
5. Ladle into soup bowls and serve.

Italian Meatballs

Serves: 6-8

Ingredients:

- ½ pound ground turkey
- 1 pound ground sirloin
- 1 egg
- ¼ teaspoon dried basil
- ½ teaspoon dried parsley
- ¼ teaspoon garlic powder
- ¼ teaspoon garlic salt
- 1 ½ teaspoons Italian seasoning
- Black pepper to taste
- 1/8 teaspoon red pepper flakes
- ½ teaspoon dried minced onions
- ¼ cup coconut flour
- A pinch paprika
- ½ teaspoon salt or to taste
- 3 cups spaghetti sauce

Method:

1. Add all the ingredients except spaghetti sauce into a mixing bowl. Mix well using your hands.
2. Shape the mixture into small meatballs of about 1 ½ inches diameter.
3. Grease a baking sheet with cooking spray. Place the meatballs on the prepared baking sheet.
4. Bake in a preheated oven at 350° F for 30 minutes or until cooked.
5. Place a skillet over medium heat. Add spaghetti sauce. Drop the meatballs in it. Stir until the meatballs are well coated with the sauce.

6. Bring to the boil. Lower heat and simmer for 10-12 minutes.
7. Serve hot or warm. Unused meatballs can be frozen in zip lock bags.

Chocolate Cupcakes with Chocolate Cashew Cream Icing

Serves: 12

Ingredients:

For the cupcakes:

- 4 large eggs
- 1 cup cocoa powder, unsweetened
- 1 teaspoon cream of tartar or 4 teaspoons baking powder
- ¼ teaspoon sea salt
- ½ cup extra virgin coconut oil
- ½ cup raw honey
- ¼ teaspoon baking soda

For the icing:

- 2 cups cashew, soaked into water for 2-3 hours, drained
- 4 tablespoons pure maple syrup
- 6 tablespoons cocoa powder, unsweetened
- 1 teaspoon vanilla extract
- ½ cup vanilla almond milk, unsweetened

Method:

1. To make cupcakes: Place 12 cupcake liners in muffin tin.
2. Add eggs, oil, cocoa, honey, salt, baking soda, cream of tartar and vanilla. Mix well but should not over- mix.
3. Pour batter into the muffin tins. Fill up to 2/3.
4. Bake in a preheated oven at 350° F for 20-30 minutes or until a toothpick when inserted in the center comes out clean.
5. Remove the cupcakes from the tin and cool completely.

6. Meanwhile make the icing as follows: Add all the ingredients of the icing into a <u>blender</u>.
7. Blend for 30-40 seconds or until smooth. Add icing into a piping bag with a star nozzle. Pipe on the top of the cupcakes.

Mini Paleo Crust Pizzas

Serves: 8

Ingredients:

For the pizza crust:

- 4 medium eggs
- 1 teaspoon salt
- 1 teaspoon dried oregano
- 2/3 cup coconut flour
- 1 1/3 cups tapioca flour
- 3 ounces butter, melted
- 1 teaspoon garlic powder
- ½ cup warm water

For the toppings:

- 4 tablespoons tomato paste
- 1 teaspoon dried oregano
- 4 tablespoons olive oil
- 2 cups Paleo cheddar cheese, grated
- 1/3 cup olives, pitted, sliced
- 2 large tomatoes, chopped
- Chili flakes to garnish

Method:

1. To make pizza crust: Add eggs, butter, water, garlic powder and oregano into a bowl. Whisk well.
2. Add Tapioca and coconut flour and mix until a thick batter is formed.

3. Line a baking sheet with parchment paper. Drop about 2-3 tablespoons of batter on the baking sheet. Using the back of a spoon lightly spread the batter to get uniform pizza crust.
4. Leave a gap between 2 crusts. Bake in batches if required or place 2 baking sheets.
5. Place in the middle rack of the oven. Bake in a preheated oven at 480° F until the crusts are light brown in color.
6. Remove the baking sheet from the oven.
7. Add tomato paste, oil and oregano into a bowl and mix well. Spread this mixture on top of the pizza crusts.
8. Sprinkle cheese. Place tomatoes and olives over it. Sprinkle red chili flakes.
9. Place the baking sheet back in the oven.
10. Reduce the temperature of the oven to 400° F. Bake for a few minutes until the cheese melts and brown in spots.
11. Serve.

Grilled Salmon Burgers with Avocado Salsa

Serves: 8

Ingredients:

<u>For burgers:</u>

- 2 pounds salmon fillets, finely chopped
- 2 eggs
- 1 poblano pepper, deseeded, chopped
- 1 teaspoon salt or to taste
- ½ teaspoon pepper or to taste
- 1 cup panko bread crumbs
- 4 green onions, thinly sliced
- 2 tablespoons fresh lemon juice or lime juice

<u>For avocado salsa:</u>

- 2 large ripe avocadoes, peeled, deseeded, chopped into small pieces
- 1 poblano pepper, deseeded, chopped
- 2 tablespoons fresh lemon juice or lime juice
- Pepper to taste
- Salt to taste
- 4 green onions, thinly sliced

Method:

1. To make avocado salsa: Add all the ingredients of avocado salsa into a bowl and stir. Cover and set aside for a while for the flavors to set in.
2. Add all the ingredients of burger into a bowl. Mix until well combined. Divide the mixture into 8 equal portions and shape into patties.

3. Cook the burgers on a preheated grill on both the sides (4 minutes per side).
4. Spoon salsa over the burgers. Serve as it is or with Paleo buns.

Paleo Pesto "Pasta" with Sausages

Serves: 4

Ingredients:

- 4 zucchinis
- ½ cup walnuts, lightly toasted
- 12 cloves garlic, peeled
- Salt to taste
- 2 red bell pepper, chopped
- 2 cups fresh basil leaves
- ½ cup almonds, lightly toasted
- 6 tablespoons extra virgin olive oil
- 2 cups spiced chicken sausage pieces

Method:

1. Make noodles of the zucchini with a spiralizer or with a julienne peeler.
2. Steam the noodles for 4-5 minutes.
3. Place a skillet over medium heat. Add about tablespoon oil. When the oil is heated, add sausages and cook until brown. Add bell pepper and sauté for a minute. Remove from heat.
4. Add walnuts, almonds, basil, garlic, salt and remaining oil into a blender. Blend until smooth.
5. To serve: Divide and place zucchini noodles on individual serving plates. Place sausage mixture over it. Drizzle pesto on top and serve.

Paleo Banana Chocolate Shake

Serves: 2

Ingredients:

- 4 bananas, peeled, sliced, frozen
- 1 cup coconut milk
- 3 teaspoons dark chocolate cocoa powder
- 1 cup cold water
- ¼ teaspoon ground cinnamon
- 2 tablespoons almond butter

Method:

1. Add all the ingredients into a <u>blender</u>. Blend for 30-40 seconds or until smooth.
2. Add more coconut milk if you want a shake of thinner consistency.

Dairy-Free Chocolate Peanut Butter Ice Cream

Serves:

Ingredients:

<u>For frozen balls:</u>

- ½ cup creamy peanut butter

<u>For the ice cream:</u>

- ½ cup honey or maple syrup
- 4 tablespoons cocoa powder, unsweetened
- 2 cans full fat coconut cream
- ½ cup peanut butter
- 2 teaspoons vanilla extract
- ½ cup peanut butter

Method:

1. Line a freezer safe dish with wax paper. Take about a teaspoon of peanut butter and drop on the wax paper. Similarly drop the remaining peanut butter.
2. Add all the ingredients of ice cream into the <u>blender</u> and blend for 30-40 seconds or until smooth.
3. Transfer into an <u>ice cream maker</u> and churn according to the manufacturer's instructions.
4. Add peanut butter balls during the last couple of minutes of churning.
5. Transfer into an airtight container and freeze until use.

Chicken Fettuccini Alfredo

Serves: 2

Ingredients:

- 4.5 ounces Cappello's gluten / grain free fettuccine, cook according to the instructions on the package, drain
- 1 shallots, minced
- 1 ½ tablespoons butter
- Sea salt to taste
- Pepper to taste
- ¼ teaspoons ground nutmeg
- 3 white mushrooms, sliced
- ½ cup Paleo friendly cheese, shredded or shaved
- 2 teaspoons olive oil, divided
- 1 chicken breast, boneless, skinless, halved
- 3 cloves garlic, minced
- ½ teaspoon pepper powder
- 1 cup Paleo whipped cream or coconut cream
- ½ cup broccoli, steamed

Method:

1. Drizzle teaspoon oil over the cooked pasta and set aside.
2. Place a skillet over medium heat. Add butter. When the butter melts, add shallots and sauté for a couple of minutes.
3. Add garlic and sauté until fragrant.
4. Add Paleo cream, nutmeg, salt and pepper and stir. Lower heat and allow it to simmer for 7-8 minutes.
5. Meanwhile, season chicken with salt and pepper and place on a preheated grill. Grill for 4 minutes on each side or until done.

6. When done, remove and place on your <u>cutting board</u>. When cool enough to handle, slice into small chunks.
7. Now add mushrooms to the simmering sauce. Simmer for a few more minutes until the mushroom is tender.
8. Add chicken, pasta and broccoli and stir. Raise the heat to medium heat. Heat thoroughly.
9. Add cheese and stir. Serve hot.

Spaghetti Squash Thai 'Noodle' Bowl

Serves: 4

Ingredients:

- 2 small spaghetti squashes
- 4 cups broccoli, steamed
- 2 tablespoons sesame seeds
- Thai peanut dressing, as required
- 4 cups water
- Sriracha sauce, as required
- 2 tablespoons sesame seeds

For Thai peanut dressing:

- 3 tablespoons honey
- 6 tablespoons vegetable oil
- 2 tablespoons tamari or soy sauce
- 2 tablespoons ginger, grated
- 4 tablespoons plain peanut butter
- 4 cloves garlic, minced
- 1 teaspoon salt
- 1 teaspoon sesame seeds (optional)
- 1 teaspoon sriracha (optional)
- 6 tablespoons rice wine vinegar
- 2 teaspoons sesame oil

Method:

1. Chop the spaghetti squash in half. Discard the seeds. Prick some holes all over the top of the spaghetti squash with a fork.
2. Add water into a large pot. Place the pot over medium heat.

95

3. Now place the squash with its cut side down.
4. Cover and cook until tender.
5. Meanwhile make the dressing as follows: Add all the ingredients of the dressing into a bowl and whisk well.
6. When done, remove the squash from the pot. Scoop out the squash using a fork and divide into bowls.
10. Place broccoli in each bowl. Drizzle the dressing over it. Garnish with sesame seeds and serve.

Chapter 8: Seven Day Meal Plan

Day 1 – Step-by-Step Video Tutorials Included

Breakfast – Almond Butter Banana Pancakes

Lunch – Celery and Asparagus Soup

Dinner - Cheesy Chicken a la Mexicana

Desserts – Chocolate Mousse with Avocado

Day 2

Breakfast - Paleo Frittata

Lunch - Roast Chicken with Veggies

Dinner - Paleo Lasagna

Desserts - Chocolate Hazelnut Balls

Day 3

Breakfast - Coconut Flour Pancakes

Lunch - Shepherd's Pie Paleo Style

Dinner - Stuffed Zucchini

Desserts - Berry and Coconut Cream Sundae

Day 4

Breakfast - Blueberry Muffins Paleo Style

Lunch - Roast Salmon

Dinner - Chicken Casserole

Desserts - Paleo Flan

Day 5

Breakfast - Paleo Dry Fruit Cereal Mix

Lunch - Turkey Burgers

Dinner - Ham and Butternut Squash Hash

Desserts - Peachy Berry Cobbler

Day 6

Breakfast - Good Health Smoothie

Lunch - Peppery Shrimps

Dinner - Baked Eggplant with Salsa

Desserts - Pumpkin Spiced Ice cream

Day 7

Breakfast – Sweet Porridge

Lunch - Grilled Pork

Dinner - Paleo Veggie Fish Bake

Desserts - Fresh Berry Mousse

Conclusion

Thank you again for downloading this book!

The Paleo Diet is an extremely healthy diet and, when it is followed to the T, you can easily knock those extra pounds off, while living a healthier and much fulfilling life!

While following the Paleo diet, you do not need to count your calories or count every ounce of nutrition that you consume. But, this does not mean that you can consume unlimited quantities of food. For example, though the Paleo diet allows the consumption of nuts, you need to make sure that you do not consume too many of them! This is because nuts have a large amount of calories and can result in increased weight if left unchecked.

Once you start following the diet, you will get a rough idea of what foods work for you and what don't! Go with your instinct and you will come up with a viable diet plan in no time at all.

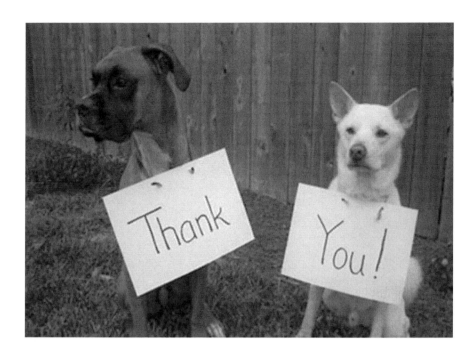

Finally, if you enjoyed this book, then I'd like to ask you for a favor, would you be kind enough to leave a review for this book on Amazon? It would be greatly appreciated!

I am trying to reach as many people as I can with this book and more reviews will help me accomplish that!

Visit the website below to leave a review for this book on Amazon!

http://amzn.to/2r432t9

FREE BONUS: **http://bit.ly/2g0mvDu**

Thank you and good luck!

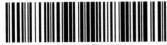

Printed in Great Britain
by Amazon